ANTI-INFLAMMATORY DIET COOKBOOK FOR VEGETARIAN

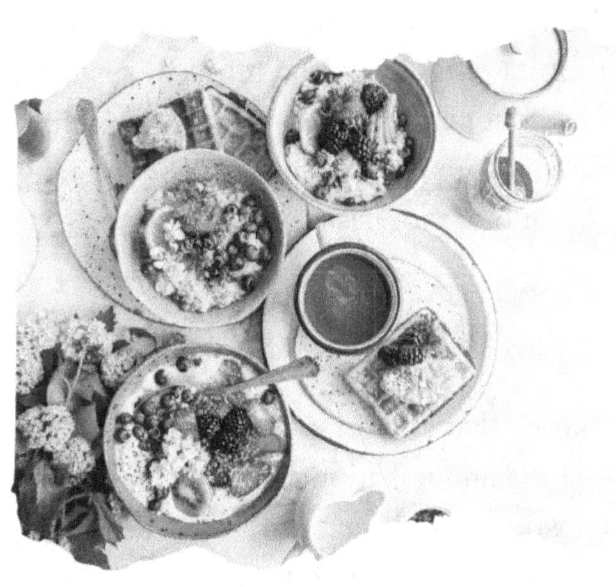

Easy To Cook Plant-based Recipes To Reduce Chronic Inflammation

KEVIN S. MAXWELL

EMAIL ME!

I know that exploring topics that involve food and nutrition can often lead to questions and uncertainty. I invite you to contact me with any questions you may have. I'm here to assist.

Please contact me through email at kevinmaxwelldiet@gmail.com, and I will try my best to respond to you within 24 hours.

Additionally, if you are interested in exploring other collections of my books. You can check out additional collections of my books by scanning the QR Code that is provided below.

HOW TO USE THIS COOKBOOK

1. Familiarize Yourself with the Cookbook:
Begin by thoroughly reading the introductory sections of the Anti-inflammatory Diet Cookbook for Vegetarians. Understand the principles of an anti-inflammatory diet, the benefits it offers, and the specific guidelines provided by the cookbook.

2. Browse and Choose Recipes:
Take time to browse through the recipe sections. Identify recipes that align with your taste preferences and dietary goals. Look for variety in ingredients and preparation methods to keep your meals exciting and nutritionally diverse.

3. Create a Weekly Meal Plan:
Plan your meals for the week by selecting a variety of recipes from the cookbook. Consider factors such as convenience, available time for preparation, and the

ingredients you already have. Creating a weekly meal plan will streamline your grocery shopping and ensure a balanced diet.

4. Prepare Ingredients in Advance:

To save time during the week, consider prepping some ingredients in advance. Chop vegetables, cook grains, and marinate proteins as needed. Having these components ready will make it easier to follow through with the recipes on busy days.

5. Enjoy and Adapt:

Follow the cookbook's recipes as closely as possible, but don't hesitate to adapt them based on personal preferences or ingredient availability. Feel free to experiment with flavors and ingredients to make the recipes truly your own. The key is to enjoy the process and savor the delicious, anti-inflammatory meals that contribute to your overall well-being.

TABLE OF CONTENT

Green Goddess Smoothie

Tropical Turmeric Smoothie

Peanut Butter Banana Protein Smoothie

Citrus Burst Smoothie

FISH AND SEAFOOD

Grilled Lemon Garlic Salmon

Shrimp and Avocado Salad

Baked Cod with Herbs

Coconut Curry Shrimp

Lemon Herb Butter Scallops

POULTRY AND MEATS

Herb-Roasted Chicken with Vegetables

Beef and Broccoli Stir-Fry

Turkey and Quinoa Stuffed Peppers

Honey Mustard Glazed Salmon

Lamb and Vegetable Skewers with Tzatziki

SALADS

Greek Salad with Tzatziki Dressing

Quinoa and Chickpea Salad

Asian Sesame Chicken Salad

Caprese Salad with Balsamic Glaze

Southwest Black Bean and Corn Salad

SOUP AND STEWS

Minestrone Soup

Moroccan Lentil Stew

Chicken and Wild Rice Soup

Butternut Squash and Apple Soup

DESSERT

Chocolate Avocado Mousse

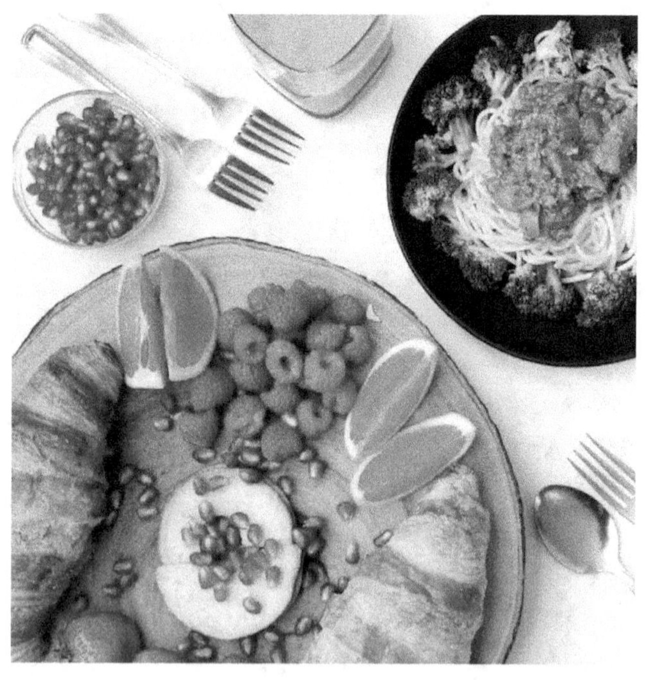

INTRODUCTION

In a quaint little town nestled between rolling hills and meandering streams, lived an old woman named Margaret. At 78, Margaret was known for her lively spirit and warm heart. However, arthritis had started to take its toll on her, causing inflammation and discomfort in her joints.

Margaret was determined to find a way to manage her inflammation without relying solely on medication. She began to explore various options and stumbled upon an anti-inflammatory diet for vegetarians. Armed with newfound knowledge, she decided to embark on a culinary journey, transforming her kitchen into a haven of healing.

She acquired an "Anti-Inflammatory Diet Cookbook for Vegetarians" and eagerly started experimenting with recipes rich in antioxidants and anti-inflammatory ingredients. Margaret spent hours poring over the pages, learning about the power of turmeric, ginger, leafy greens, and other wholesome foods that could help alleviate inflammation.

Her mornings began with a warm cup of turmeric tea, and her days were filled with colorful salads, vibrant stir-fries, and nourishing soups. Margaret marveled at the variety of flavors and textures she could create using plant-based ingredients. She sourced fresh produce from the local farmers' market, fostering a connection with the community and the earth.

As weeks passed, Margaret noticed a remarkable change in her health. The stiffness in her joints began to subside, and she felt more agile and energetic. Her friends and neighbors couldn't help but marvel at the transformation, and soon, Margaret became the go-to person for advice on healthy living.

One sunny afternoon, Margaret decided to share her newfound passion with the community. She invited her friends and neighbors to a delightful vegetarian feast prepared entirely from recipes in her anti-inflammatory cookbook. The aroma of roasted vegetables, lentil curry, and quinoa salad filled the air as laughter and joy echoed through Margaret's home.

As everyone savored the delicious, healing dishes, Margaret shared her journey and the positive impact of embracing an anti-inflammatory vegetarian diet. Inspired by her story, many in the community decided to adopt healthier eating habits, creating a ripple effect of well-being.

Margaret's kitchen became a hub of culinary exploration and communal support. The anti-inflammatory diet not only brought relief to her arthritis but also forged stronger connections within the community. Margaret, the spirited old woman with a heart full of warmth, had not only found a way to manage her inflammation but had also sown the seeds of health and happiness for those around her.

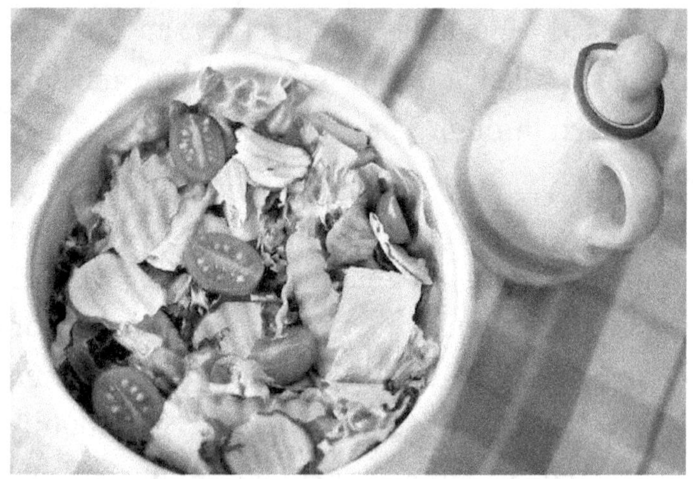

CHAPTER 1: WHAT IS ANTI-INFLAMMATORY DIET

The anti-inflammatory diet is centered around consuming foods that help reduce inflammation in the body, promoting overall health and potentially preventing or managing certain chronic conditions. Chronic inflammation has been linked to various health issues, including heart disease, arthritis, and some types of cancer. The goal of the anti-inflammatory diet is to include foods with anti-inflammatory properties while minimizing those that may contribute to inflammation.

Key Principles of an Anti-Inflammatory Diet

1. Fruits and Vegetables: Rich in antioxidants and phytochemicals, fruits and vegetables play a crucial role in an anti-inflammatory diet. Berries, leafy greens, tomatoes, and cruciferous vegetables are excellent choices.

2. Whole Grains: Opt for whole grains such as brown rice, quinoa, and oats, which provide fiber and nutrients.

3. Healthy Fats: Include sources of healthy fats, such as olive oil, avocados, and nuts, which have anti-inflammatory properties.

4. Fatty Fish: Fatty fish like salmon, mackerel, and sardines are high in omega-3 fatty acids, known for their anti-inflammatory effects.

5. Legumes: Beans, lentils, and chickpeas are rich in fiber and protein and are associated with anti-inflammatory benefits.

6. Herbs and Spices: Turmeric, ginger, garlic, and other herbs and spices have anti-inflammatory properties and can be incorporated into meals.

7. Limit Processed Foods: Processed and refined foods, as well as those high in added sugars and unhealthy fats, can contribute to inflammation. Minimize their consumption.

8. Moderate Alcohol: If consumed, do so in moderation, as excessive alcohol intake can contribute to inflammation.

An anti-inflammatory diet cookbook for vegetarians focuses on providing plant-based recipes that align with the principles of the anti-inflammatory diet. These cookbooks often include creative and flavorful recipes using a variety of vegetables, fruits, whole grains, legumes, and plant-based proteins. They may also incorporate herbs and spices known for their anti-inflammatory properties, such as turmeric, ginger, and cinnamon.

EFFECT OF THE INFLAMMATION ON THE BODY

Inflammation is a natural and essential part of the body's immune response. It is a complex biological process that occurs in response to injury, infection, or tissue damage. While acute inflammation is a protective mechanism that helps the body heal and defend against harmful invaders, chronic inflammation can have detrimental effects on the body. Here's an overview of the effects of inflammation on the body:

1. Immune System Activation:
Inflammation involves the activation of the immune system, including the release of white blood cells and signaling molecules called cytokines. These immune responses are crucial for eliminating pathogens and initiating tissue repair.

2. Increased Blood Flow:

Blood vessels in the affected area dilate during inflammation, leading to increased blood flow. This brings more immune cells, oxygen, and nutrients to the site of injury or infection.

3. Heat and Redness:

Increased blood flow contributes to heat and redness in the inflamed area, indicating an influx of immune cells and heightened metabolic activity.

4. Swelling:

The accumulation of fluid and immune cells can lead to swelling, which helps isolate the damaged area and protect surrounding tissues.

5. Pain:

Inflammation can stimulate nerve endings, resulting in pain or discomfort. Pain serves as a signal that something is wrong and helps prevent further damage.

6. Fever:

In response to certain infections or inflammatory triggers, the body may elevate its temperature (fever). Fever can enhance the immune response and inhibit the growth of some pathogens.

7. Tissue Damage Repair:

Acute inflammation is a critical part of the healing process, facilitating the removal of damaged cells and tissues and promoting the regeneration of new, healthy tissue.

However, when inflammation becomes chronic or persists for an extended period, it can lead to harmful effects:

1. Tissue Damage and Fibrosis:

Prolonged inflammation can cause damage to healthy tissues, leading to fibrosis (scarring). This can impair the normal function of organs and tissues.

2. Autoimmune Diseases:

In some cases, the immune system mistakenly targets and attacks healthy cells and tissues, leading to autoimmune diseases. Conditions like rheumatoid arthritis, lupus, and psoriasis are examples of autoimmune disorders characterized by chronic inflammation.

3. Chronic Diseases:

Chronic inflammation has been linked to the development and progression of various chronic diseases, including cardiovascular diseases, type 2 diabetes, and certain cancers.

4. Impact on Mental Health:

Emerging research suggests a potential connection between chronic inflammation and mental health disorders, including depression and anxiety.

Managing inflammation through lifestyle choices, such as adopting a healthy diet, regular exercise, stress management, and

adequate sleep, is crucial for preventing or mitigating the harmful effects of chronic inflammation. It's essential to seek medical advice for persistent or severe inflammation, as it may indicate underlying health conditions that require professional evaluation and treatment.

DISEASES RELATED TO INFLAMMATION

Chronic inflammation has been linked to various diseases and health conditions. While inflammation is a natural and necessary part of the body's immune response to injury or infection, chronic or prolonged inflammation can contribute to the development and progression of several diseases. Here are some diseases that are associated with inflammation:

1. Cardiovascular Diseases:

Chronic inflammation is a contributing factor to the development of atherosclerosis, a condition where the arteries become narrowed and hardened due to the buildup of plaque. This can lead to heart attacks and strokes.

2. Rheumatoid Arthritis:

An autoimmune disorder where the immune system mistakenly attacks the joints, causing

inflammation, pain, and swelling. Chronic inflammation in the joints can lead to joint damage and deformities.

3. Inflammatory Bowel Diseases (IBD):

Conditions such as Crohn's disease and ulcerative colitis involve chronic inflammation of the gastrointestinal tract, leading to symptoms like abdominal pain, diarrhea, and weight loss.

4. Type 2 Diabetes:

Chronic low-grade inflammation is associated with insulin resistance, a key factor in the development of type 2 diabetes. Inflammation may interfere with normal insulin function and glucose regulation.

5. Cancer:

Chronic inflammation has been linked to the development of certain cancers. Inflammation can promote the growth of tumors and contribute to the progression of cancer.

6. Neurodegenerative Diseases:

Conditions like Alzheimer's and Parkinson's diseases are associated with chronic inflammation in the brain. Inflammation may contribute to the degeneration of nerve cells and the progression of these disorders.

7. Chronic Obstructive Pulmonary Disease (COPD):

Inflammatory changes in the airways and lungs are common in COPD, a group of lung diseases that includes chronic bronchitis and emphysema.

8. Psoriasis:

A chronic skin condition characterized by red, itchy, and scaly patches. It is an autoimmune disease involving inflammation in the skin.

9. Systemic Lupus Erythematosus (SLE):

An autoimmune disease where the immune system attacks various organs and tissues, leading to inflammation and damage.

10. Gout:

A type of arthritis caused by the buildup of uric acid crystals in the joints, leading to inflammation and severe pain.

It's important to note that while inflammation is implicated in the development of these conditions, it may not be the sole cause. Genetics, lifestyle factors, and environmental influences also play significant roles. Managing inflammation through a healthy lifestyle, including a balanced diet, regular exercise, and stress management, can contribute to overall well-being and may help prevent or manage certain inflammatory-related diseases. Individuals with specific health concerns should consult with healthcare professionals for personalized advice and treatment.

UNDERSTANDING INFLAMMATION

Inflammation is a natural and essential part of the body's immune response to injury or infection. It involves the activation of the immune system to repair damaged tissues, fight off pathogens, and promote healing. While acute inflammation is a normal and protective process, chronic inflammation can be harmful and is linked to various health conditions.

Types of Inflammation

1. Acute Inflammation: This is a short-term, localized response to injury or infection. It involves the rapid activation of immune cells, increased blood flow, and the release of substances that help eliminate the cause of cell injury.

2. Chronic Inflammation: This is a prolonged and sustained inflammatory response that can last for weeks, months, or even years. Chronic inflammation is associated with various diseases, including rheumatoid arthritis, cardiovascular disease, and some types of cancer.

Symptoms of Inflammation

Common symptoms of inflammation include:

- Redness
- Swelling
- Heat
- Pain
- Loss of function in the affected area

These symptoms can vary depending on the type of inflammation and its underlying cause.

Preventive Measures for Inflammation

1. Maintain a Healthy Diet: Consuming a well-balanced diet rich in fruits, vegetables, whole grains, and lean proteins can help reduce inflammation. Certain foods, such as fatty fish (rich in omega-3 fatty acids), turmeric, and ginger, are known for their anti-inflammatory properties.

2. Regular Exercise: Engaging in regular physical activity can help modulate the inflammatory response. Exercise has been shown to have anti-inflammatory effects and contributes to overall health.

3. Adequate Sleep: Lack of sleep or poor sleep quality can contribute to inflammation. Ensuring sufficient and quality sleep is crucial for maintaining overall well-being.

4. Stress Management: Chronic stress can trigger inflammation. Practices such as meditation, yoga, and deep breathing exercises can help manage stress and reduce inflammation.

5. Avoiding Smoking and Excessive Alcohol Consumption: Both smoking and excessive alcohol intake can contribute to inflammation and negatively impact health. Quitting smoking and moderating alcohol consumption are essential for preventing inflammation-related issues.

6. Regular Health Check-ups: Regular medical check-ups can help identify and address potential health issues early, preventing the development of chronic inflammation.

It's important to note that individual responses to inflammation can vary, and any persistent or severe symptoms should be discussed with a healthcare professional for proper evaluation and guidance.

CHAPTER 2: BENEFITS OF ANTI-INFLAMMATORY DIET

Adopting an anti-inflammatory diet can offer various health benefits by focusing on foods that help reduce inflammation in the body.

Here are some core benefits of following an anti-inflammatory diet:

1. Reduced Chronic Inflammation:

The primary goal of an anti-inflammatory diet is to mitigate chronic inflammation. By emphasizing foods with anti-inflammatory properties, such as fruits, vegetables, and fatty fish, and reducing the intake of pro-inflammatory foods, the diet aims to lower overall inflammation levels in the body.

2. Improved Heart Health:

Chronic inflammation is a contributing factor to cardiovascular diseases. An anti-inflammatory diet that includes heart-healthy foods like fatty fish, nuts, and olive oil can help lower the risk of heart disease by reducing inflammation and improving lipid profiles.

3. Joint Health and Arthritis Management:

Individuals with arthritis, particularly rheumatoid arthritis, may benefit from an anti-inflammatory diet. Foods rich in omega-3 fatty acids, antioxidants, and anti-inflammatory spices can help manage joint pain and stiffness.

4. Balanced Blood Sugar Levels:

An anti-inflammatory diet, which often includes whole grains, fruits, and vegetables, can contribute to better blood sugar control. This is beneficial for individuals with or at risk of type 2 diabetes.

5. Weight Management:

Maintaining a healthy weight is crucial for preventing inflammation. An anti-inflammatory diet that includes nutrient-dense, whole foods and limits processed and sugary foods can support weight management and reduce inflammation associated with obesity.

6. Improved Gut Health:

The anti-inflammatory diet promotes a diverse range of fruits, vegetables, and fiber-rich foods, which can positively impact gut health. A healthy gut microbiome is associated with reduced inflammation and improved overall well-being.

7. Enhanced Immune Function:

Nutrient-rich foods in an anti-inflammatory diet, such as fruits, vegetables, and lean proteins, provide essential vitamins and minerals that support a robust immune system. A well-functioning immune system helps the body defend against infections and diseases.

8. Cancer Prevention:

While no diet can guarantee cancer prevention, an anti-inflammatory diet rich in antioxidants and phytochemicals may help reduce the risk of certain cancers. These foods can neutralize free radicals and support the body's natural defense mechanisms.

9. Improved Mental Health:

There is growing evidence suggesting a link between inflammation and mental health conditions. An anti-inflammatory diet, along with other lifestyle factors, may positively influence mood and reduce the risk of depression and anxiety.

10. Anti-Aging Benefits:

Chronic inflammation is associated with aging and age-related diseases. By reducing inflammation, an anti-inflammatory diet may contribute to healthy aging and support longevity.

CHAPTER 3: TIPS TO ACHIEVE OPTIMAL HEALTH WITH ANTI-INFLAMMATORY DIET

Adopting an anti-inflammatory diet, especially with a focus on vegetarian options, can significantly contribute to achieving optimum health. An anti-inflammatory diet emphasizes whole, nutrient-dense foods while minimizing processed and pro-inflammatory choices. Let's explore the foods to include and avoid in a vegetarian anti-inflammatory diet, drawing insights from an Anti-Inflammatory Diet Cookbook for Vegetarians.

Foods to Eat

1. Colorful Fruits and Vegetables:
Rich in antioxidants, vitamins, and minerals, fruits and vegetables are staples in an anti-inflammatory diet. Berries, leafy

greens, tomatoes, and bell peppers provide a spectrum of phytochemicals that combat inflammation.

2. Whole Grains:

Opt for whole grains such as brown rice, quinoa, oats, and whole wheat. These grains contain fiber and essential nutrients, contributing to stable blood sugar levels and reducing inflammation.

3. Healthy Fats:

Incorporate sources of healthy fats, including avocados, nuts, seeds, and olive oil. These fats are rich in omega-3 fatty acids and monounsaturated fats, known for their anti-inflammatory properties.

4. Fatty Fish Alternatives:

While many anti-inflammatory diets include fatty fish, vegetarians can choose plant-based sources of omega-3s, such as chia seeds, flaxseeds, and walnuts, to support heart and brain health.

5. Legumes:

Beans, lentils, chickpeas, and other legumes are excellent sources of protein, fiber, and various anti-inflammatory compounds. They also contribute to gut health by promoting a diverse microbiome.

6. Herbs and Spices:

Herbs and spices like turmeric, ginger, garlic, and cinnamon have potent anti-inflammatory and antioxidant properties. Incorporate these flavorful additions to enhance the taste of dishes while promoting health.

7. Plant-Based Proteins:

Include plant-based protein sources such as tofu, tempeh, and edamame. These alternatives provide protein without the saturated fats found in some animal products.

8. Dairy Alternatives:

Choose dairy alternatives like almond milk, coconut milk, or soy milk. These options can be fortified with essential nutrients and may be suitable for those with lactose intolerance or seeking plant-based alternatives.

Foods to Limit or Avoid

1. Processed Foods:

Minimize the consumption of processed and refined foods, as they often contain additives, preservatives, and unhealthy fats that may contribute to inflammation.

2. Added Sugars:

Reduce intake of added sugars found in sugary beverages, sweets, and processed snacks. Excessive sugar consumption can contribute to inflammation and negatively impact overall health.

3. Refined Grains:

Limit the intake of refined grains like white bread and white rice, as they lack the fiber and nutrients present in whole grains.

4. Saturated and Trans Fats:

Avoid sources of saturated and trans fats, commonly found in fried foods, certain oils, and some processed snacks. These fats can contribute to inflammation and raise cholesterol levels.

5. Excessive Omega-6 Fatty Acids:

While omega-6 fatty acids are essential, an imbalance with omega-3s can promote inflammation. Reduce consumption of oils high in omega-6, such as corn and soybean oil.

6. Highly Processed Meat Alternatives:

Some vegetarian meat alternatives can be highly processed and contain additives. Opt for whole food sources of protein like legumes and tofu rather than heavily processed substitutes.

7. Artificial Additives and Preservatives:

Choose whole, minimally processed foods over those containing artificial additives and preservatives, as these substances may contribute to inflammation in some individuals.

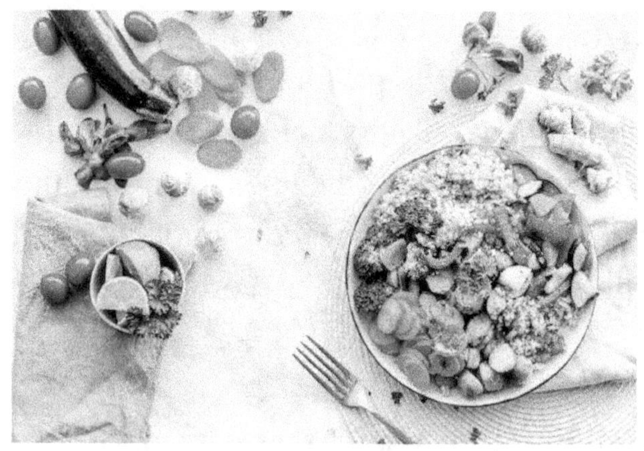

CHAPTER 4: ANTI-INFLAMMATORY RECIPES

BREAKFAST AND BRUNCH

Berry and Almond Overnight Oats

Ingredients:
- Rolled oats (1 cup)
- Almond milk (1 cup)
- Mixed berries (1/2 cup, fresh or frozen)
- Almonds (2 tbsp, sliced)
- Chia seeds (1 tbsp)
- Maple syrup (1 tbsp)
- Vanilla extract (1/2 tsp)

Instructions:
1. In a jar or container, combine rolled oats, almond milk, mixed berries, sliced almonds, chia seeds, maple syrup, and vanilla extract.

2. Stir well to ensure all ingredients are evenly distributed.
3. Seal the jar or container and refrigerate overnight.
4. In the morning, give the mixture a good stir and add extra almond milk if desired.
5. Top with additional berries and almonds before serving.

Avocado and Tomato Breakfast Toast

Ingredients:
- Whole-grain bread slices (2)
- Avocado (1, mashed)
- Cherry tomatoes (1/2 cup, sliced)
- Red onion (2 tbsp, finely chopped)
- Fresh cilantro (2 tbsp, chopped)
- Lime juice (1 tbsp)
- Salt and pepper to taste

Instructions:

1. Toast the whole-grain bread slices to your liking.
2. In a bowl, combine mashed avocado, sliced cherry tomatoes, chopped red onion, fresh cilantro, lime juice, salt, and pepper.
3. Spread the avocado mixture evenly over the toasted bread slices.
4. Garnish with extra cilantro and a dash of black pepper before serving.

Spinach and Mushroom Frittata

Ingredients:

- Eggs (4)
- Spinach leaves (1 cup, chopped)
- Mushrooms (1/2 cup, sliced)
- Red bell pepper (1/4 cup, diced)
- Feta cheese (1/4 cup, crumbled)
- Olive oil (1 tbsp)
- Salt and pepper to taste

Instructions:

1. Preheat the oven to 350°F (180°C).
2. In an oven-safe skillet, sauté mushrooms and red bell pepper in olive oil until softened.
3. Add chopped spinach and cook until wilted.
4. In a bowl, whisk eggs and season with salt and pepper.
5. Pour the egg mixture over the vegetables in the skillet.
6. Sprinkle crumbled feta cheese on top.
7. Bake for 15-20 minutes or until the frittata is set and slightly golden.
8. Slice and serve warm.

Quinoa and Berry Parfait

Ingredients:

- Cooked quinoa (1 cup)
- Greek yogurt (1/2 cup)
- Mixed berries (1/2 cup, fresh or frozen)
- Honey (1 tbsp)

- Almonds (2 tbsp, chopped)
- Vanilla extract (1/2 tsp)

Instructions:
1. In a glass or bowl, layer cooked quinoa, Greek yogurt, and mixed berries.
2. Drizzle honey over the layers.
3. Sprinkle chopped almonds on top.
4. Repeat the layers if desired.
5. Finish with a splash of vanilla extract.
6. Enjoy immediately as a refreshing and nutrient-packed parfait.

Sweet Potato and Black Bean Breakfast Burrito

Ingredients:
- Sweet potato (1, medium, cooked and mashed)
- Black beans (1/2 cup, cooked)
- Whole-grain tortilla (1)
- Avocado (1/2, sliced)
- Salsa (2 tbsp)

- Fresh cilantro (1 tbsp, chopped)
- Lime wedge (1)
- Salt and pepper to taste

Instructions:

1. In a bowl, mix mashed sweet potato and cooked black beans.
2. Season with salt and pepper.
3. Warm the whole-grain tortilla in a dry skillet or microwave.
4. Spread the sweet potato and black bean mixture onto the tortilla.
5. Top with sliced avocado, salsa, and chopped cilantro.
6. Squeeze lime juice over the filling.
7. Fold the sides of the tortilla and roll it into a burrito.
8. Serve warm and enjoy a satisfying and flavorful breakfast.

Berry Bliss Smoothie

Ingredients:

- Mixed berries (1 cup, fresh or frozen)
- Banana (1, frozen)
- Greek yogurt (1/2 cup)
- Almond milk (1 cup)
- Chia seeds (1 tbsp)
- Honey (1 tbsp, optional for sweetness)

Instructions:

1. Combine mixed berries, frozen banana, Greek yogurt, almond milk, chia seeds, and honey (if desired) in a blender.
2. Blend until smooth and creamy.
3. Pour into a glass and enjoy this antioxidant-rich berry smoothie.

Green Goddess Smoothie

Ingredients:

- Spinach leaves (1 cup)
- Pineapple chunks (1/2 cup, frozen)
- Mango (1/2 cup, frozen)
- Avocado (1/4)
- Coconut water (1 cup)
- Fresh mint leaves (a handful)

Instructions:

1. Place spinach leaves, frozen pineapple chunks, frozen mango, avocado, coconut water, and fresh mint leaves in a blender.
2. Blend until the mixture reaches a smooth consistency.
3. Pour into a glass and savor the refreshing taste of this green smoothie.

Tropical Turmeric Smoothie

Ingredients:

- Pineapple (1 cup, fresh or frozen)
- Mango (1/2 cup, frozen)
- Banana (1, frozen)
- Turmeric powder (1/2 tsp)
- Ginger (1/2 tsp, grated)
- Coconut milk (1 cup)

Instructions:

1. Combine pineapple, frozen mango, frozen banana, turmeric powder, grated ginger, and coconut milk in a blender.
2. Blend until all ingredients are well combined.
3. Pour into a glass and enjoy the tropical and anti-inflammatory goodness of this smoothie.

Peanut Butter Banana Protein Smoothie

Ingredients:

- Banana (1, frozen)
- Peanut butter (2 tbsp)
- Greek yogurt (1/2 cup)
- Almond milk (1 cup)
- Vanilla protein powder (1 scoop)
- Ice cubes (optional)

Instructions:

1. In a blender, combine frozen banana, peanut butter, Greek yogurt, almond milk, vanilla protein powder, and ice cubes if desired.
2. Blend until the smoothie reaches a creamy consistency.
3. Pour into a glass for a protein-packed and satisfying smoothie.

Citrus Burst Smoothie

Ingredients:

- Oranges (2, peeled and segmented)
- Pineapple (1 cup, fresh or frozen)
- Strawberries (1/2 cup, fresh or frozen)
- Greek yogurt (1/2 cup)
- Almond milk (1 cup)
- Ice cubes (optional)

Instructions:

1. Place orange segments, pineapple, strawberries, Greek yogurt, almond milk, and ice cubes (if desired) in a blender.
2. Blend until the mixture is smooth and citrusy.
3. Pour into a glass and relish the refreshing taste of this citrus burst smoothie.

Grilled Lemon Garlic Salmon

Ingredients:

- Salmon fillets (4, skin-on)
- Garlic cloves (3, minced)
- Lemon (1, juiced)
- Olive oil (3 tbsp)
- Dijon mustard (1 tbsp)
- Fresh dill (2 tbsp, chopped)
- Salt and black pepper to taste

Instructions:

1. In a bowl, whisk together minced garlic, lemon juice, olive oil, Dijon mustard, chopped dill, salt, and pepper.
2. Place salmon fillets in a shallow dish and pour the marinade over them. Let it marinate for at least 30 minutes.
3. Preheat the grill to medium-high heat.
4. Grill salmon fillets for 4-5 minutes per side or until cooked through.

5. Serve with additional lemon wedges and garnish with fresh dill.

Shrimp and Avocado Salad

Ingredients:
- Shrimp (1 lb, peeled and deveined)
- Avocado (2, diced)
- Cherry tomatoes (1 cup, halved)
- Red onion (1/4 cup, finely chopped)
- Cilantro (2 tbsp, chopped)
- Lime (1, juiced)
- Olive oil (2 tbsp)
- Salt and black pepper to taste

Instructions:
1. In a large bowl, combine shrimp, diced avocado, cherry tomatoes, chopped red onion, and cilantro.
2. In a small bowl, whisk together lime juice, olive oil, salt, and black pepper.
3. Pour the dressing over the shrimp and avocado mixture and toss gently to coat.

4. Chill in the refrigerator for at least 30 minutes before serving.

Baked Cod with Herbs

Ingredients:
- Cod fillets (4)
- Lemon (1, sliced)
- Fresh parsley (3 tbsp, chopped)
- Fresh dill (2 tbsp, chopped)
- Garlic powder (1 tsp)
- Olive oil (3 tbsp)
- Salt and black pepper to taste

Instructions:
1. Preheat the oven to 400°F (200°C).
2. Place cod fillets in a baking dish and season with salt, black pepper, and garlic powder.
3. Drizzle olive oil over the fillets and sprinkle chopped parsley and dill on top.
4. Arrange lemon slices on and around the cod.

5. Bake for 15-20 minutes or until the fish flakes easily with a fork.

Coconut Curry Shrimp

Ingredients:
- Shrimp (1 lb, peeled and deveined)
- Coconut milk (1 can)
- Red curry paste (2 tbsp)
- Bell peppers (2, sliced)
- Zucchini (1, sliced)
- Onion (1, sliced)
- Garlic (3 cloves, minced)
- Ginger (1 tbsp, grated)
- Fish sauce (2 tbsp)
- Fresh cilantro (2 tbsp, chopped)
- Cooked rice for serving

Instructions:
1. In a pan, heat coconut milk over medium heat.
2. Stir in red curry paste, minced garlic, and grated ginger.

3. Add shrimp, bell peppers, zucchini, and onion to the pan.
4. Simmer until shrimp are cooked through and vegetables are tender.
5. Stir in fish sauce and sprinkle with fresh cilantro.
6. Serve over cooked rice.

Lemon Herb Butter Scallops

Ingredients:
- Scallops (1 lb)
- Lemon (1, juiced)
- Fresh thyme (1 tbsp, chopped)
- Fresh parsley (2 tbsp, chopped)
- Unsalted butter (3 tbsp)
- Garlic (2 cloves, minced)
- Salt and black pepper to taste

Instructions:
1. Pat the scallops dry with paper towels and season with salt and black pepper.
2. In a skillet, melt butter over medium heat.

3. Add minced garlic and sauté for 1-2
   minutes.
4. Add scallops to the skillet and cook
   for 2-3 minutes per side or until
   golden brown.
5. Drizzle with lemon juice and sprinkle
   with chopped thyme and parsley
   before serving.

Herb-Roasted Chicken with Vegetables

Ingredients:
- Whole chicken (4-5 lbs)
- Potatoes (1 lb, diced)
- Carrots (1 lb, sliced)
- Onion (1, sliced)
- Garlic cloves (4, minced)
- Fresh rosemary (2 tbsp, chopped)
- Fresh thyme (2 tbsp, chopped)
- Olive oil (3 tbsp)
- Salt and black pepper to taste

Instructions:
1. Preheat the oven to 425°F (220°C).
2. In a bowl, mix chopped rosemary, thyme, minced garlic, olive oil, salt, and black pepper.
3. Rub the herb mixture over the chicken and place it in a roasting pan.
4. Arrange diced potatoes, sliced carrots, and sliced onion around the chicken.

5. Roast for 1 to 1.5 hours or until the chicken is cooked through and vegetables are tender.

Beef and Broccoli Stir-Fry

Ingredients:
- Beef sirloin or flank steak (1 lb, thinly sliced)
- Broccoli florets (3 cups)
- Soy sauce (1/4 cup)
- Oyster sauce (2 tbsp)
- Sesame oil (1 tbsp)
- Garlic (3 cloves, minced)
- Ginger (1 tbsp, grated)
- Brown sugar (2 tbsp)
- Vegetable oil (2 tbsp)
- Cooked rice for serving

Instructions:
1. In a bowl, whisk together soy sauce, oyster sauce, sesame oil, minced garlic, grated ginger, and brown sugar.

2. Heat vegetable oil in a wok or skillet over high heat.
3. Add thinly sliced beef and stir-fry until browned.
4. Add broccoli to the wok and continue stir-frying until the broccoli is tender-crisp.
5. Pour the sauce over the beef and broccoli, tossing to coat evenly. Serve over cooked rice.

Turkey and Quinoa Stuffed Peppers

Ingredients:

- Bell peppers (4, halved and seeds removed)
- Ground turkey (1 lb)
- Quinoa (1 cup, cooked)
- Black beans (1/2 cup, canned and drained)
- Corn kernels (1/2 cup, fresh or frozen)
- Tomato sauce (1 cup)
- Chili powder (1 tsp)
- Cumin (1 tsp)

- Shredded cheddar cheese (1/2 cup)
- Fresh cilantro (2 tbsp, chopped)

Instructions:

1. Preheat the oven to 375°F (190°C).
2. In a skillet, cook ground turkey until browned. Drain excess fat.
3. In a bowl, mix cooked quinoa, black beans, corn, tomato sauce, chili powder, and cumin.
4. Stuff bell peppers with the turkey mixture and place them in a baking dish.
5. Top each stuffed pepper with shredded cheddar cheese.
6. Bake for 25-30 minutes or until the peppers are tender.
7. Garnish with chopped fresh cilantro before serving.

Honey Mustard Glazed Salmon

Ingredients:
- Salmon fillets (4)
- Dijon mustard (2 tbsp)
- Honey (2 tbsp)
- Soy sauce (1 tbsp)
- Garlic powder (1 tsp)
- Olive oil (2 tbsp)
- Lemon wedges for serving

Instructions:
1. Preheat the oven to 400°F (200°C).
2. In a bowl, whisk together Dijon mustard, honey, soy sauce, garlic powder, and olive oil.
3. Place salmon fillets in a baking dish and brush the glaze over each fillet.
4. Bake for 12-15 minutes or until the salmon is cooked through.
5. Serve with lemon wedges.

Lamb and Vegetable Skewers with Tzatziki

Ingredients:

- Lamb cubes (1 lb)
- Bell peppers (2, diced)
- Red onion (1, diced)
- Cherry tomatoes (1 cup)
- Olive oil (3 tbsp)
- Garlic (3 cloves, minced)
- Lemon juice (2 tbsp)
- Dried oregano (1 tsp)
- Salt and black pepper to taste
- Wooden skewers (pre-soaked in water)
- Tzatziki sauce for dipping

Instructions:

1. In a bowl, mix olive oil, minced garlic, lemon juice, dried oregano, salt, and black pepper.
2. Thread lamb cubes, bell peppers, red onion, and cherry tomatoes onto the soaked wooden skewers.

3. Brush the skewers with the olive oil mixture.

4. Grill the skewers over medium-high heat for 10-12 minutes, turning occasionally, until the lamb is cooked to your liking.

5. Serve with tzatziki sauce for dipping.

Greek Salad with Tzatziki Dressing

Ingredients:
- Cherry tomatoes (1 cup, halved)
- Cucumber (1, diced)
- Kalamata olives (1/2 cup, pitted)
- Red onion (1/4 cup, thinly sliced)
- Feta cheese (1/2 cup, crumbled)
- Mixed greens (4 cups)
- Tzatziki dressing:
- Greek yogurt (1/2 cup)
- Lemon juice (2 tbsp)
- Garlic (1 clove, minced)
- Fresh dill (1 tbsp, chopped)
- Salt and black pepper to taste

Instructions:
1. In a large bowl, combine cherry tomatoes, cucumber, Kalamata olives, red onion, feta cheese, and mixed greens.

2. In a separate bowl, whisk together Greek yogurt, lemon juice, minced garlic, chopped fresh dill, salt, and black pepper to create the tzatziki dressing.
3. Pour the dressing over the salad and toss gently to coat.
4. Serve immediately, and enjoy the vibrant flavors of this Greek-inspired salad.

Quinoa and Chickpea Salad

Ingredients:
- Cooked quinoa (2 cups)
- Chickpeas (1 can, drained and rinsed)
- Cherry tomatoes (1 cup, halved)
- Cucumber (1, diced)
- Red bell pepper (1, diced)
- Red onion (1/4 cup, finely chopped)
- Feta cheese (1/2 cup, crumbled)
- Fresh parsley (2 tbsp, chopped)
- Olive oil (3 tbsp)
- Lemon juice (2 tbsp)

- Salt and black pepper to taste

Instructions:
1. In a large bowl, combine cooked quinoa, chickpeas, cherry tomatoes, cucumber, red bell pepper, red onion, and feta cheese.
2. In a small bowl, whisk together olive oil, lemon juice, salt, and black pepper to create the dressing.
3. Pour the dressing over the salad and toss gently.
4. Garnish with chopped fresh parsley before serving.

Asian Sesame Chicken Salad

Ingredients:
- Chicken breast (1, grilled and sliced)
- Mixed salad greens (4 cups)
- Carrots (2, julienned)
- Red cabbage (1 cup, thinly sliced)
- Edamame (1/2 cup, cooked)
- Cucumber (1, thinly sliced)

- Sesame seeds (2 tbsp)
- Green onions (2 tbsp, chopped)
- Sesame ginger dressing:
- Soy sauce (2 tbsp)
- Rice vinegar (2 tbsp)
- Sesame oil (1 tbsp)
- Honey (1 tbsp)
- Ginger (1 tsp, grated)

Instructions:

1. In a large bowl, combine grilled and sliced chicken breast, mixed salad greens, julienned carrots, thinly sliced red cabbage, edamame, cucumber, sesame seeds, and chopped green onions.

2. In a small bowl, whisk together soy sauce, rice vinegar, sesame oil, honey, and grated ginger to create the dressing.

3. Pour the dressing over the salad and toss gently.

4. Serve immediately, and enjoy the Asian-inspired flavors.

Caprese Salad with Balsamic Glaze

Ingredients:

- Tomatoes (2, sliced)
- Fresh mozzarella cheese (1 ball, sliced)
- Fresh basil leaves (1 cup)
- Balsamic glaze (2 tbsp)
- Extra virgin olive oil (2 tbsp)
- Salt and black pepper to taste

Instructions:

1. Arrange sliced tomatoes, fresh mozzarella cheese, and fresh basil leaves on a serving platter.
2. Drizzle balsamic glaze and extra virgin olive oil over the salad.
3. Season with salt and black pepper to taste.
4. Serve immediately as a classic and refreshing Caprese salad.

Southwest Black Bean and Corn Salad

Ingredients:

- Black beans (1 can, drained and rinsed)
- Corn kernels (1 cup, fresh or frozen, cooked)
- Cherry tomatoes (1 cup, halved)
- Avocado (1, diced)
- Red onion (1/4 cup, finely chopped)
- Fresh cilantro (2 tbsp, chopped)
- Lime juice (2 tbsp)
- Olive oil (2 tbsp)
- Cumin (1 tsp)
- Chili powder (1/2 tsp)
- Salt and black pepper to taste

Instructions:

1. In a large bowl, combine black beans, cooked corn kernels, cherry tomatoes, diced avocado, finely chopped red onion, and chopped fresh cilantro.
2. In a small bowl, whisk together lime juice, olive oil, cumin, chili powder,

salt, and black pepper to create the dressing.

3. Pour the dressing over the salad and toss gently.

4. Serve chilled, and enjoy the vibrant flavors of this Southwest-inspired salad.

Minestrone Soup

Ingredients:
- Olive oil (2 tbsp)
- Onion (1, diced)
- Carrots (2, diced)
- Celery (2 stalks, diced)
- Garlic (3 cloves, minced)
- Crushed tomatoes (1 can, 14 oz)
- Cannellini beans (1 can, drained and rinsed)
- Vegetable broth (6 cups)
- Zucchini (1, diced)
- Green beans (1 cup, chopped)
- Pasta (1/2 cup, small shape)
- Spinach (2 cups, chopped)
- Italian seasoning (1 tsp)
- Salt and black pepper to taste
- Parmesan cheese (for garnish)

Instructions:

1. In a large pot, heat olive oil over medium heat. Sauté onion, carrots, celery, and garlic until softened.
2. Add crushed tomatoes, cannellini beans, vegetable broth, zucchini, green beans, pasta, Italian seasoning, salt, and black pepper.
3. Simmer for 15-20 minutes or until the vegetables and pasta are tender.
4. Stir in chopped spinach and cook until wilted.
5. Serve hot, garnished with Parmesan cheese.

Moroccan Lentil Stew

Ingredients:

- Olive oil (2 tbsp)
- Onion (1, diced)
- Carrots (2, diced)
- Red lentils (1 cup, rinsed)
- Sweet potato (1, peeled and diced)
- Vegetable broth (4 cups)

- Ground cumin (1 tsp)
- Ground coriander (1 tsp)
- Paprika (1/2 tsp)
- Ground cinnamon (1/2 tsp)
- Cayenne pepper (1/4 tsp, optional)
- Salt and black pepper to taste
- Fresh cilantro (for garnish)

Instructions:

1. In a large pot, heat olive oil over medium heat. Sauté onion and carrots until softened.
2. Add red lentils, sweet potato, vegetable broth, cumin, coriander, paprika, cinnamon, cayenne pepper (if using), salt, and black pepper.
3. Bring to a boil, then reduce heat and simmer for 25-30 minutes or until lentils and sweet potatoes are tender.
4. Adjust seasoning if necessary and serve hot, garnished with fresh cilantro.

Chicken and Wild Rice Soup

Ingredients:

- Chicken breasts (2, boneless and skinless)
- Wild rice (1 cup, uncooked)
- Carrots (3, diced)
- Celery (3 stalks, diced)
- Onion (1, diced)
- Garlic (3 cloves, minced)
- Chicken broth (6 cups)
- Thyme (1 tsp, dried)
- Bay leaves (2)
- Butter (2 tbsp)
- All-purpose flour (1/4 cup)
- Heavy cream (1 cup)
- Salt and black pepper to taste
- Fresh parsley (for garnish)

Instructions:

1. In a large pot, combine chicken breasts, wild rice, carrots, celery, onion, garlic, chicken broth, thyme, and bay leaves.

2. Bring to a boil, then reduce heat and simmer until chicken is cooked through and rice is tender.
3. Remove chicken, shred it, and return to the pot.
4. In a separate pan, melt butter, whisk in flour, and cook for 1-2 minutes.
5. Slowly whisk in heavy cream until smooth, then add the mixture to the soup.
6. Season with salt and black pepper. Discard bay leaves.
7. Serve hot, garnished with fresh parsley.

Butternut Squash and Apple Soup

Ingredients:
- Butternut squash (1, peeled and diced)
- Apples (2, peeled, cored, and diced)
- Onion (1, diced)
- Vegetable broth (4 cups)
- Coconut milk (1 can, 13.5 oz)

- Curry powder (1 tsp)
- Ground nutmeg (1/2 tsp)
- Cinnamon (1/2 tsp)
- Olive oil (2 tbsp)
- Salt and black pepper to taste
- Pumpkin seeds (for garnish)

Instructions:

1. In a large pot, heat olive oil over medium heat. Sauté onion until softened.
2. Add butternut squash, apples, vegetable broth, coconut milk, curry powder, nutmeg, and cinnamon.
3. Bring to a boil, then reduce heat and simmer until squash and apples are tender.
4. Use an immersion blender to puree the soup until smooth.
5. Season with salt and black pepper. Serve hot, garnished with pumpkin seeds.

Chocolate Avocado Mousse

Ingredients:
- Avocados (2, ripe)
- Cocoa powder (1/2 cup)
- Maple syrup (1/4 cup)
- Vanilla extract (1 tsp)
- Almond milk (1/4 cup)
- Pinch of salt
- Fresh berries (for garnish)

Instructions:
1. In a blender, combine ripe avocados, cocoa powder, maple syrup, vanilla extract, almond milk, and a pinch of salt.
2. Blend until smooth and creamy.
3. Chill in the refrigerator for at least 1 hour.
4. Serve the chocolate avocado mousse in individual bowls, garnished with fresh berries.

Raspberry Lemon Bars

Ingredients:

- Butter (1 cup, softened)
- Granulated sugar (1/2 cup)
- All-purpose flour (2 cups)
- Eggs (4)
- Lemon juice (1/2 cup)
- Raspberry jam (1/2 cup)
- Powdered sugar (for dusting)

Instructions:

1. Preheat the oven to 350°F (180°C) and grease a baking dish.
2. In a bowl, cream together softened butter, granulated sugar, and flour.
3. Press the mixture into the prepared baking dish to form the crust.
4. Bake for 15-20 minutes or until the edges are golden.
5. In another bowl, whisk together eggs and lemon juice. Pour over the baked crust.
6. Drop small spoonfuls of raspberry jam on top.

7. Bake for an additional 25-30 minutes or until the filling is set.

8. Allow to cool, then dust with powdered sugar before cutting into bars.

Coconut Chia Pudding

Ingredients:
- Coconut milk (1 can, 13.5 oz)
- Chia seeds (1/2 cup)
- Maple syrup (2 tbsp)
- Vanilla extract (1 tsp)
- Shredded coconut (2 tbsp, toasted)
- Fresh mango slices (for topping)

Instructions:
1. In a bowl, whisk together coconut milk, chia seeds, maple syrup, and vanilla extract.
2. Let the mixture sit for 30 minutes, stirring occasionally.
3. Refrigerate for at least 2 hours or overnight until it thickens.

4. Toast shredded coconut in a dry pan until golden brown.
5. Serve the coconut chia pudding in individual bowls, topped with toasted coconut and fresh mango slices.

Apple Cinnamon Crisp

Ingredients:

- Apples (4, peeled, cored, and sliced)
- Lemon juice (1 tbsp)
- Granulated sugar (1/4 cup)
- Ground cinnamon (1 tsp)
- All-purpose flour (1 tbsp)
- Oats (1 cup)
- Brown sugar (1/2 cup, packed)
- Butter (1/2 cup, melted)
- Vanilla ice cream (for scrving)

Instructions:

1. Preheat the oven to 350°F (180°C) and grease a baking dish.

2. In a bowl, toss sliced apples with lemon juice, granulated sugar, ground cinnamon, and flour.
3. In another bowl, mix oats, brown sugar, and melted butter to create the crisp topping.
4. Spread the apple mixture in the baking dish and sprinkle the crisp topping over it.
5. Bake for 40-45 minutes or until the top is golden and the apples are tender.
6. Allow to cool slightly before serving with a scoop of vanilla ice cream.

Pistachio and Rosewater Semolina Cake

Ingredients:
- Semolina (1 cup)
- Pistachios (1/2 cup, finely ground)
- Baking powder (1 tsp)
- Butter (1/2 cup, softened)
- Granulated sugar (1/2 cup)

- Eggs (3)
- Yogurt (1/2 cup)
- Rosewater (1 tbsp)
- Powdered sugar (for dusting)

Instructions:

1. Preheat the oven to 350°F (180°C) and grease a cake pan.
2. In a bowl, whisk together semolina, ground pistachios, and baking powder.
3. In another bowl, cream together softened butter and granulated sugar.
4. Add eggs one at a time, beating well after each addition.
5. Stir in yogurt and rosewater.
6. Gradually add the dry ingredients to the wet ingredients, mixing until well combined.
7. Pour the batter into the prepared cake pan and smooth the top.
8. Bake for 25-30 minutes or until a toothpick inserted into the center comes out clean.

9. Allow the cake to cool, then dust with
    powdered sugar before serving.

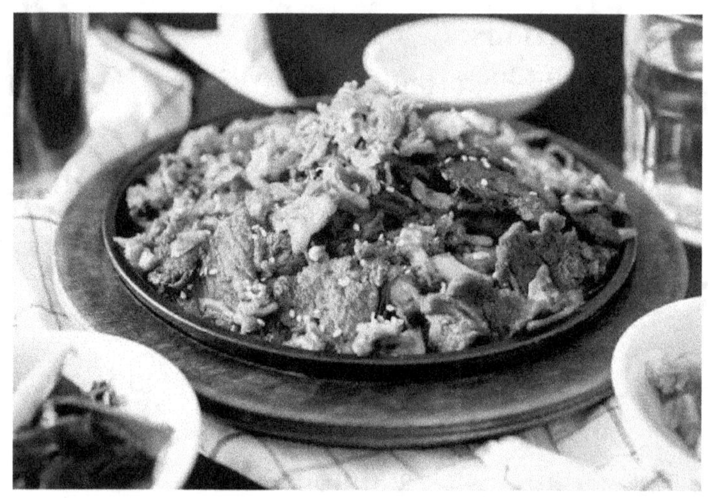

CHAPTER 5: MEAL PLANNING

HOW TO USE THE MEAL PLAN

1. Review the Meal Plan:

Take a moment to review the 14-day anti-inflammatory diet meal plan. Familiarize yourself with the recipes for each day, including breakfast, lunch, and dinner.

2. Create a Shopping List:

Based on the meal plan, compile a shopping list with all the necessary ingredients for the recipes. Check your pantry and fridge to see if you already have some items. Ensure you have everything you need for the next two weeks.

3. Prep Ingredients in Advance:

To make meal preparation easier, consider doing some prep work in advance. Wash and chop vegetables, cook grains, and marinate proteins as needed. Store these prepped items in containers to streamline the cooking process during the week.

4. Rotate Recipes and Customize:
While following the meal plan, feel free to rotate recipes based on your preferences. If there's a particular recipe you enjoyed, you can repeat it later in the week. Additionally, customize the plan to accommodate any dietary restrictions or personal preferences.

5. Stay Hydrated and Listen to Your Body:
Alongside the provided meals, remember to stay hydrated by drinking plenty of water throughout the day. Listen to your body's hunger and fullness cues, and adjust portion sizes or snack options accordingly. If you have specific health concerns or dietary needs, consult with a healthcare professional or a registered dietitian for personalized guidance.

14-DAY MEAL PLAN

Day 1:

Breakfast: Berry and Almond Overnight Oats
Lunch: Quinoa and Chickpea Salad
Dinner: Grilled Lemon Garlic Salmon with Mediterranean Stuffed Acorn Squash

Day 2:

Breakfast: Avocado and Tomato Breakfast Toast
Lunch: Greek Salad with Tzatziki Dressing
Dinner: Moroccan Lentil Stew

Day 3:

Breakfast: Spinach and Mushroom Frittata
Lunch: Quinoa and Berry Parfait
Dinner: Baked Cod with Herbs

Day 4:

Breakfast: Peanut Butter Banana Protein Smoothie
Lunch: Southwest Black Bean and Corn Salad
Dinner: Coconut Curry Shrimp

Day 5:

Breakfast: Citrus Burst Smoothie
Lunch: Caprese Salad with Balsamic Glaze
Dinner: Lemon Herb Butter Scallops

Day 6:

Breakfast: Berry Bliss Smoothie
Lunch: Chicken and Wild Rice Soup
Dinner: Quinoa and Chickpea Salad

Day 7:

Breakfast: Sweet Potato and Black Bean Breakfast Burrito
Lunch: Butternut Squash and Apple Soup

Dinner: Grilled Lemon Garlic Salmon with Mediterranean Stuffed Acorn Squash

Day 8:

Breakfast: Avocado and Tomato Breakfast Toast
Lunch: Greek Salad with Tzatziki Dressing
Dinner: Moroccan Lentil Stew

Day 9:

Breakfast: Spinach and Mushroom Frittata
Lunch: Quinoa and Berry Parfait
Dinner: Baked Cod with Herbs

Day 10:

Breakfast: Peanut Butter Banana Protein Smoothie
Lunch: Southwest Black Bean and Corn Salad
Dinner: Coconut Curry Shrimp

Day 11:

Breakfast: Citrus Burst Smoothie
Lunch: Caprese Salad with Balsamic Glaze
Dinner: Lemon Herb Butter Scallops

Day 12:

Breakfast: Berry Bliss Smoothie
Lunch: Chicken and Wild Rice Soup
Dinner: Quinoa and Chickpea Salad

Day 13:

Breakfast: Sweet Potato and Black Bean
Breakfast Burrito
Lunch: Butternut Squash and Apple Soup
Dinner: Grilled Lemon Garlic Salmon with
Mediterranean Stuffed Acorn Squash

Day 14:

Breakfast: Avocado and Tomato Breakfast Toast
Lunch: Greek Salad with Tzatziki Dressing
Dinner: Moroccan Lentil Stew

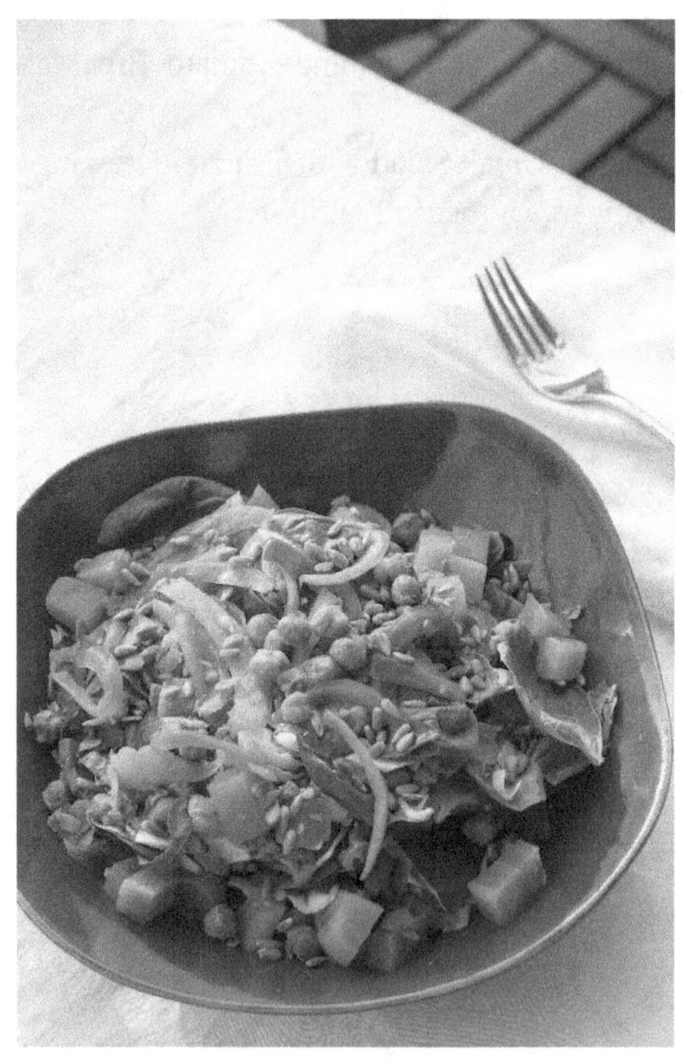

CONCLUSION

In conclusion, the Anti-inflammatory Diet Cookbook for Vegetarian not only offers a delectable array of recipes but also serves as a comprehensive guide to fostering well-being through mindful nutrition. With a focus on plant-based ingredients rich in antioxidants and anti-inflammatory properties, this cookbook empowers readers to make health-conscious choices that support overall vitality.

The diverse range of recipes, from Mediterranean Stuffed Acorn Squash to Quinoa and Chickpea Salad, provides a delightful journey into the world of vegetarian culinary excellence. As you embark on this transformative dietary path, remember that adopting and adapting to the anti-inflammatory diet is not just a culinary choice but a pledge towards long-term health.

Make this commitment your personal journey toward well-being, embracing the delicious flavors and nourishing ingredients that will leave you feeling energized, satisfied, and motivated on the road to a healthier, more vibrant lifestyle.

Thank you for this invaluable Anti-inflammatory Diet Cookbook for Vegetarian. The diverse and delicious recipes, combined with insightful guidance, have empowered me to make mindful and health-conscious choices. Grateful for this transformative culinary journey towards well-being.

BONUS: WEEKLY MEAL PLANNER JOURNAL

MEAL PLANNER

Weekly

WEEK

MONTH

MONDAY

SATURDAY

TUESDAY

SUNDAY

WEDNESDAY

SHOPPING LIST

THURSDAY

FRIDAY

MEAL PLANNER

Weekly

WEEK _______________   MONTH _______________

MONDAY

TUESDAY

WEDNESDAY

THURSDAY

FRIDAY

SATURDAY

SUNDAY

SHOPPING LIST

MEAL PLANNER

Weekly

WEEK ___________________

MONTH ___________________

MONDAY

TUESDAY

WEDNESDAY

THURSDAY

FRIDAY

SATURDAY

SUNDAY

SHOPPING LIST

MEAL PLANNER

Weekly

WEEK ______________________   MONTH ______________________

MONDAY

SATURDAY

TUESDAY

SUNDAY

WEDNESDAY

SHOPPING LIST

THURSDAY

FRIDAY

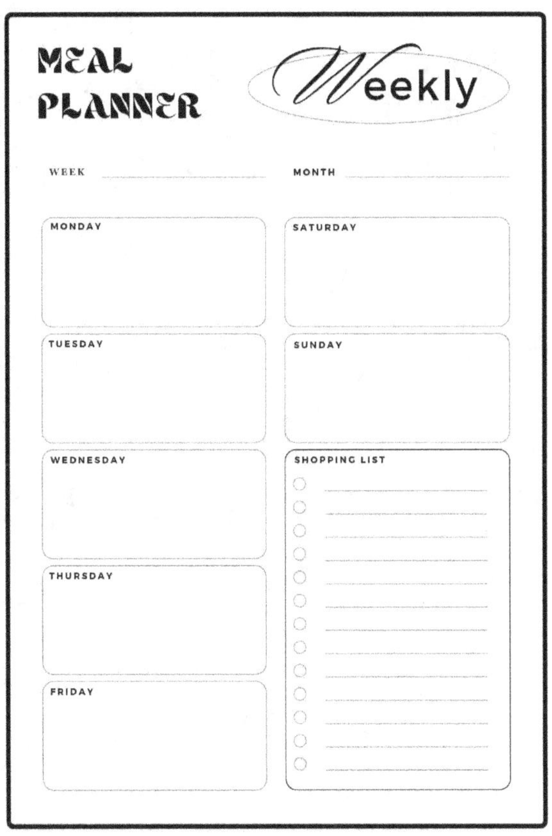

MEAL PLANNER
Weekly
WEEK
MONTH
MONDAY
SATURDAY
TUESDAY
SUNDAY
WEDNESDAY
SHOPPING LIST
THURSDAY
FRIDAY

MEAL PLANNER

Weekly

WEEK ______________________   MONTH ______________________

MONDAY

TUESDAY

WEDNESDAY

THURSDAY

FRIDAY

SATURDAY

SUNDAY

SHOPPING LIST

MEAL PLANNER

Weekly

WEEK __________________   MONTH __________________

MONDAY

TUESDAY

WEDNESDAY

THURSDAY

FRIDAY

SATURDAY

SUNDAY

SHOPPING LIST

MEAL PLANNER

Weekly

WEEK ______________________   MONTH ______________________

MONDAY

SATURDAY

TUESDAY

SUNDAY

WEDNESDAY

SHOPPING LIST

-
-
-
-
-
-
-
-
-
-
-

THURSDAY

FRIDAY

MEAL PLANNER

Weekly

WEEK ___________________   MONTH ___________________

MONDAY

SATURDAY

TUESDAY

SUNDAY

WEDNESDAY

THURSDAY

FRIDAY

SHOPPING LIST

MEAL PLANNER

Weekly

WEEK ________________   MONTH ________________

MONDAY

TUESDAY

WEDNESDAY

THURSDAY

FRIDAY

SATURDAY

SUNDAY

SHOPPING LIST

www.ingramcontent.com/pod-product-compliance
Lightning Source LLC
Chambersburg PA
CBHW070832260726
48660CB00005B/2021